John F. Reynolds, PhD

THE CANCER CODE

The Complete Guide on How to Starve Cancer Without Starving

Table of Contents

Preface

The word "cancer" is wide. It explains the illness that develops as a consequence of unchecked cell growth and division brought on by cellular alterations. While certain cancer types cause cells to grow and divide more slowly than others, other cancer types promote fast cell proliferation.

While certain cancers, like leukemia, may not cause visible growths known as tumors, others, like carcinoma, do.

The majority of cells in the body have set purposes and lifespans. Although it may seem harmful, cell death is a normal and advantageous process known as apoptosis.

A cell is given the go-ahead to pass away so that the body may swap it out with a younger, more functional cell.

Cancerous cells are deficient in the elements that tell healthy cells to cease proliferating and to die.

As a consequence, they accumulate throughout the body and consume nutrients and oxygen that would otherwise feed other cells. Tumors, immune system impairment, and other changes brought on by cancerous cells may prohibit the body from operating normally.

The lymph nodes may allow cancerous cells to spread from where they first appeared. Immune cell colonies may be seen throughout the body.

Cancer is genetic?

The onset of cancer may be influenced by genetic factors.

The genetic coding of a person determines when their cells will divide and die. Gene changes may result in incorrect instructions, which may cause cancer.

Proteins contain many of the instructions for cellular development and division, and genes may also affect how proteins are produced by the cells.

Certain genes alter the proteins that would typically mend harmed cells. This could result in cancer. The changed instructions might be passed on to a child if a parent has these genes.

Some genetic alterations may place after birth, and risks might be increased by things like smoking and sun exposure.

The chemical signals that control how the body uses, or "expresses," certain genes undergo other alterations that might result in cancer.

Finally, a propensity to a certain form of cancer might be inherited. This can be referred to as having a hereditary cancer syndrome by a doctor. A considerable portion of cancer cases (5–10%) is caused by inherited genetic alterations.

Part One: The Beast

Volume 1: Understanding Metabolism Protocol

The alteration of intracellular signaling pathways caused by mutant oncogenes and tumor-suppressor genes directly affects the metabolism of cancer cells. Oncogenic gene mutations may start the metabolism of cancer cells right away. Similarly, altered metabolic enzymes may promote the development of cancer. Cells benefit from metabolism, an energy-producing process, for maintaining cell homeostasis as well as for growth and proliferation.

To sense environmental signals and run metabolic machinery to supply enough energy for life in a precisely regulated way, normal cells are equipped with intricate signaling networks that are managed by critical regulatory enzymes. To accommodate increased adenosine triphosphate (ATP) consumption for cell reproduction, normal cells engage metabolic pathways during proliferation. Reactive oxygen species are unpleasant byproducts of aerobic metabolism that, along with this metabolic boost, may harm cells and encourage DNA mutations. Therefore, changes in cell metabolism might lead to the development of tumors. Oncogene and tumor-suppressor gene mutations may change a variety of intracellular signaling pathways, which in turn alters cell metabolism to promote tumorigenesis. Changes in signaling pathways not only help cells adjust to the metabolism of tumor cells, but some of these metabolic changes are also necessary for malignant transformation.

Aerobic glycolysis, often known as the Warburg effect and named for Otto Warburg who originally characterized it in 1926, is the distinctive metabolic signature of tumor metabolism. Even under aerobic circumstances, cancer cells primarily make energy through increased glycolysis in the cytosol as opposed to normal cells, which mostly oxidize pyruvate in the mitochondria. Whether they are under normoxic or hypoxic conditions, the majority of cancer cells employ glycolysis to produce energy. It has been shown time and time again that glycolytic ATP generation and tumor aggressiveness are related. Initially, it was thought that these metabolic alterations were caused by damage to mitochondrial oxidative phosphorylation, which implied that cancer cells were unable to respire correctly to produce enough ATP.

Recent research, however, has shown that many cancer cells can synthesize ATP through mitochondrial respiration. Cancer cells still show significant rates of glycolysis and lactate fermentation regardless of whether mitochondrial respiration is decreased, and this reliance on glucose use may be exploited for therapeutic intervention.

Reprogramming of the metabolism: The Warburg effect

The major source of energy and the principal fuel for cellular respiration is glucose. It is known that 70% of the ATP required for glucose use is produced by oxidative phosphorylation, and the remaining 30% via glycolysis. The ratio of glycolysis to oxidative phosphorylation changes in various cells, growth phases, and microenvironments, just as the ATP output varies with cellular circumstances.

For instance, under hypoxia, increased glycolysis makes up for impaired oxidative phosphorylation to maintain the cellular energy balance. Despite having a functioning oxidative phosphorylation apparatus, the majority of solid tumor cells transform their metabolism from respiration to glycolysis, which manifests as cancer-specific aerobic glycolysis.

Other processes, such as lactate fermentation, are enlisted to meet the cellular energy need when the oxidative phosphorylation machinery is constrained for whatever cause (hypoxia, inhibition of mitochondrial respiration, etc.). To multiply, cancer cells need a tremendous quantity of energy in a short amount of time. When the oxygen supply is restricted or when the growth rate exceeds the usual energy supply, respectively, muscle cells in hypoxic situations and embryo cells during development may adapt to altered metabolism.

These cells need a lot of glucose, which is converted to lactate for quick but ineffective ATP synthesis. The Warburg effect describes how cancer cells also show altered metabolism to fulfill their energy requirements as the tumor progresses.

Numerous investigations have shown that metabolic changes to glucose provide extra energy to encourage tumor development. As a consequence, tumor development and cell proliferation are inhibited by glycolysis. Additionally, the suppression of glycolysis-related metabolic pathways slows the development of tumors. These indicate that inhibiting glycolysis may be an effective way to delay or halt the growth of cancer.

Cancer-related Metabolic Gene Mutations

The Warburg effect explains abnormal cancer metabolism, but mutations in the genes that make metabolic enzymes may directly relate the altered metabolism to a particular gene. A subgroup of human malignancies with mutations in two TCA cycle-related genes that encode fumarate hydratase (FH) and succinate dehydrogenase (SDH) accumulate their corresponding substrates, fumarate, and succinate.

In the electron transport chain, SDH also functions as respiratory complex II; as a result, mutations in SDH may have a direct impact on mitochondrial respiration. Indeed, hereditary paragangliomas and pheochromocytomas have been linked to mutations in the genes producing SDH subunits. The enzyme that changes fumarate into malate in the mitochondria is also encoded by the FH gene. Fumarate hydratase deficit is the outcome of FH mutations, which have also been linked to papillary kidney carcinoma, uterine and cutaneous leiomyomas, and fumarate hydratase deficiency.

A metabolic enzyme mutation has been linked to carcinogenesis, according to research on cancer genome sequencing. Isocitrate dehydrogenases IDH1 and IDH2, which are NADP (nicotinamide adenine dinucleotide phosphate)-dependent, provide an intriguing example of a mutant metabolic enzyme causing cancer. In human cells, IDH1 and IDH2 catalyze the creation of one NADPH molecule while converting isocitrate to -ketoglutarate (KG). Homodimeric enzymes IDH1 and IDH2 function in the cytoplasm and mitochondria, respectively.

In gliomas and acute myeloid leukemia, heterozygous point mutations in several IDH1 residues be frequent. The cytoplasmic KG concentration is decreased, prolyl hydroxylase activity is inhibited, and the hypoxia-induced transcription factor HIF-1 is stabilized as a result of these mutations acting in a dominant-negative manner to reduce IDH1 and IDH2 activity. Additionally, it has been shown that these mutations provide IDH1 and IDH2 new enzymatic activity, converting KG to 2-hydroxyglutarate (2-HG), with unknown consequences. Even though 2-HG is only present in trace amounts in healthy cells and tissues, mutations in IDH1 and IDH2 cause 2-HG levels in glioma tissues and acute myeloid leukemia cells to rise.

It would thus be intriguing to learn if elevated 2-HG concentrations are correlated with the tumorigenicity of IDH1 and IDH2 mutations. It's significant to note that levels of KG, isocitrate, and several other TCA metabolites are unaffected in cells or tissues with IDH1 mutations, indicating that alternative metabolic pathways may regulate

and maintain typical levels of important metabolites.

This page was left blank intentionally

This page was left blank intentionally

Volume 2: What You Need to Know

Cancer is the unchecked spread of aberrant cells throughout the body. Cancer cells, malignant cells, or tumor cells are names for these aberrant cells. These cells can invade healthy bodily tissues. The name of the tissue from which the aberrant cells originated helps to further identify many tumors and the abnormal cells that make up the cancer tissue (for example, breast cancer, lung cancer, and colorectal cancer).

Animals and other living things may also get cancer; it is not only a disease that affects people. The diagram that follows illustrates normal cell division and how, in the absence of systemic healing, a damaged or changed cell typically dies. It is also shown what happens when such injured or unrepaired cells do not perish but instead develop into cancer cells with unchecked proliferation and growth—a mass of cancer cells. Cancer cells often separate from this initial clump of cells, move through the blood and lymphatic systems, and settle in other organs where they may restart the unchecked development cycle.

Metastatic spread or metastasis refers to the process through which cancer cells leave one part of the body and spread to another. For instance, if breast cancer cells have metastasized to the bone, the patient has this condition. The term "bone cancer" is not the same thing since it would imply that the disease began in the bone.

The expected numbers of new cases and fatalities for each prevalent cancer type are shown in the following table (National Cancer Institute 2022):

Cancer	Estimated New cases	Estimated Deaths
Bladder	76,960	76,960
Breast (Female --	287,850 - 2,710	287,850 - 2,710

Male)		
Colon and Rectal (Combined)	151,030	151,030
Endometrial	65,950	65,950
Kidney (Renal Cell and Renal Pelvis) Cancer	79,000	79,000
Leukemia (All Types)	60,650	60,650
Lung (Including Bronchus)	236,740	236,740
Melanoma	99,780	43,250 - 530
Non-Hodgkin Lymphoma	80,470	52,580
Pancreatic	62,210	12,550
Prostate	268,490	13,920
Thyroid	43,800	24,000

In the United States, the top three malignancies affecting men, women, and children are as follows:

• Males: colorectal, lung, and prostate

Breast, lung, and colorectal cancer in women

• Childhood lymphoma, brain tumors, and leukemia

Numerous variables, including age, gender, race, local environmental conditions, food, and genetics, have an impact on the occurrence of cancer and the different forms of cancer. As a result, these varying variables have an impact on both the incidence of cancer and the forms of cancer. The World Health Organization (WHO), for instance, offers the general knowledge below regarding cancer globally:

The top cause of death in the world is cancer. According to the most current WHO statistics, it was responsible for 8.2 million fatalities, or around 22% of all deaths that were not caused by infectious illnesses.

• The greatest cancer-related fatalities each year are caused by breast, colon, liver, stomach, and lung cancer.

• It is anticipated that there would be 13.1 million cancer-related deaths globally in 2030, which would represent a 70% increase.

There may be malignancies that are more or less common in certain parts of the globe than in the United States. For instance, although stomach cancer is uncommon in the United States, it is often seen there. This often denotes a confluence of hereditary and environmental variables.

This book goal is to provide the reader with some basic information on cancers. It can't cover every form of cancer since it is just meant to provide an overview. Additionally, this site will make an effort to direct readers to publications that go into greater information concerning certain cancer kinds.

What are the causes and risk factors for cancer?

Any factor that might lead to an aberrant body cell's development is possibly carcinogenic. Cell abnormalities and the development of cancer have been related to a variety of causes. While some cancers have unidentified origins, others have environmental or lifestyle triggers or may have many recognized causes. Some traits may be altered by a person's genetic makeup throughout development. Combinations of these causes often result in cancer development in people.

Research has given clinicians several likely causes that, either alone or in combination with other causes, are the likely candidates for initiating cancer. This is true even though it is frequently difficult or impossible to pinpoint the initiating event(s) that lead to cancer developing in a specific person. Major reasons are listed below, however, this list is not exhaustive since new factors are often added as research progresses.

exposure to hazardous or chemical compounds: N-nitrosamines, tobacco or cigarette smoke (contains at least 66 recognized probable carcinogenic compounds and toxins), asbestos, nickel, cadmium, vinyl chloride, benzidine, and aflatoxin are just a few of the substances that might cause cancer.

Ionizing radiation is present in uranium, radon, sunlight's ultraviolet rays, as well as radiation from sources that generate alpha, beta, gamma, and X-rays.

Human papillomavirus (HPV), Epstein-Barr virus (EBV), hepatitis B and C, Merkel cell polyomavirus (KSHV), Schistosoma species, and Helicobacter pylori are pathogens; additional microorganisms are being investigated as potential culprits.

Genetics: The following malignancies have been specifically related to human genes: To learn more about the precise genes and other facts relating to breast, ovarian, colorectal, prostate, skin, and melanoma, the reader is directed to the National Cancer Institute.

It is crucial to note that while most people have cancer risk factors and are exposed to cancer-causing agents throughout their lifetime (such as sunshine, secondhand smoking, and X-rays), many people do not end up getting the disease. Additionally, a lot of individuals have genes related to cancer but do not get it. Why? It is obvious that the greater the number or level of cancer-causing elements a person is exposed to, the higher the probability the person will acquire cancer. However, researchers may not be able to provide a suitable solution for every individual.

Additionally, those with genetic predispositions to cancer may not get it for the same reasons (lack of enough stimulus to make the genes function). Additionally, some individuals may have an immune response that is more active than usual, controlling or eliminating cells that are or may develop into cancer cells. There is evidence that even certain food habits may have a big impact on whether cancer cells survive or not while working with the immune system. Due to these factors, it might be difficult to pinpoint the exact etiology of cancer in many cases.

The list of things that may raise the risk of cancer has recently been expanded to include more risk factors. The International Agency for Research on Cancer specifically designated processed foods (such as salted, smoked, preserved, and/or cured meats) as carcinogenic and red meat (such as cattle, lamb, and hog) as a high-risk agent for possibly causing malignancies.

Due to the chemicals that are created at high temperatures, those who consume a lot of grilled meat may also be at higher risk. Obesity, inactivity, persistent inflammation, and hormones, particularly those used in replacement treatment, are additional, less well-defined risk factors for certain malignancies. Numerous studies have been conducted on other things like mobile phones. Mobile phones are at the same risk as coffee and pickled vegetables according to the World Health Organization's classification of cell phone low-energy radiation as "probably carcinogenic" in 2011. However, this is a very low-risk threshold.

It might be challenging to demonstrate that a chemical is not responsible for or connected to a higher risk of developing cancer. For instance, although some researchers believe antiperspirants may be linked to breast cancer, others do not. The NCI's stated position is that "further study is required to examine this link and other potential contributing variables." The conflicting evidence gathered up to this point has led to the presentation of this unsatisfactory conclusion. Similar assertions need an extensive and costly study that may never be conducted.

Although it could be difficult to follow in complicated, technologically sophisticated contemporary civilizations, reasonable advice might be to avoid huge doses of any substances even slightly associated with cancer.

Cancer symptoms and indicators vary depending on the kind of cancer, its location, and/or the extent of the cancer cells' dissemination. Breast cancer, for instance, might show symptoms such as a lump in the breast or nipple discharge, whereas metastatic breast cancer can show signs such as discomfort (if it has spread to the bones), excessive exhaustion (lungs), or seizures (brain). Only after the cancer is far advanced do some people exhibit any signs or symptoms.

The American Cancer Society lists seven symptoms or warning signs that should cause a person to seek medical assistance if they suspect they may have cancer.

Your memory of them may be aided by the word CAUTION.

• Modifications to bowel or bladder habits

• Chronic sore throat;

• Unusual bleeding or discharge (for example, nipple secretions or a "sore" that will not heal that oozes material)

• An increase in size or a bump in the testicles, breast, or another area

• A wart or mole that has visibly changed in size, color, form, or thickness, which is often chronic

• Recurrent coughing or hoarseness

Who treats cancer in these fields?

An oncologist is a physician who focuses on the treatment of cancer. He or she could be a surgeon, radiation oncologist, or medical oncologist. In the first, cancer is treated surgically; in the second, with radiation therapy; and in the third, with chemotherapy and allied therapies. To create a treatment strategy for the specific patient, each party may speak with the others.

Depending on the location of the tumor, more doctors can be engaged. For instance, ob-gyn doctors would treat uterine cancer, but an immunologist might handle tumors that affect the immune system.

You may choose which experts would be the greatest additions to your treatment team with the assistance of your primary care physician and primary oncologist.

This page was left blank intentionally

Part 2: Healing

This page was left blank intentionally

Volume 3: Beat Cancer Mindset

Since I started my journey, I've read about, met, and interviewed many people who have healed all types and stages of cancer, and I've seen that same mindset in every single one of them. I call it the Beat Cancer Mindset. This mindset is the single most important factor, the linchpin in every successful healing story.

The Beat Cancer Mindset has five components:

1. Accept total responsibility for your health.

2. Be willing to do whatever it takes.

3. Take massive action.

4. Make plans for the future.

5. Enjoy your life and the process.

Accept total responsibility for your health.

The first question on a cancer patient's mind after diagnosis is "Why did this happen to me? How did I get cancer?"

My intention is not to blame you or shame you but to empower you to take control of your situation and change your life.

Many of the cancer-causing factors in your life can be removed and your risk of getting a recurrence or dying from cancer can be greatly reduced, just by your choices. Your choices matter. People who care about you are going to tell you the truth. Sometimes the truth stings a little, but the truth will set you free.

Accepting responsibility for your health starts with considering the possibility that cancer may be your fault.

Maybe some bad decisions, bad habits, or ignorance throughout your life contributed to your cancer. I know mine did. There's no need to beat yourself up about it or wallow in guilt, self-pity, or regret.

Instead now is the time to evaluate your life, accept whatever part you played, and learn from your mistakes. Now is the time to identify the cancer causes in your life, radically change, and move forward.

One of the most troubling things I've ever heard a cancer patient say is, "I'm not going to let cancer change me."

On the surface, this proclamation of defiance of the disease gives the impression of strength, determination, and willpower and could easily serve as a rallying cry for cancer fighters, but tragically, it is denial and disempowerment in disguise.

It was a denial that she had contributed in any way to her situation, and it was an acknowledgment that she did not believe she had the power to affect her health and her future. She did not survive. And the gravity of her statement still haunts me. Denial is far more dangerous than blaming yourself. Accepting the blame is taking responsibility.

Taking responsibility for your circumstance empowers you to take control of your life and to change for the better.

Every day in cancer clinics all over the world, patients are told that their cancer is probably the result of bad luck or bad genes.

This turns patients into victims. The logic is simple: nothing you did caused or contributed to your disease; therefore, there is nothing you can do to reverse it. If you have a family history, they may tell you it's genetic. If you don't have any family history, they may still tell you it's genetic.

Heredity and genetics are easy scapegoats, but fewer than 5 percent of cancers are genetic, and not everyone with a "cancer gene" develops cancer. Genes may load the gun, but your diet, lifestyle, and environment pull the trigger. However, if you believe that you are powerless and that there is nothing you can do to positively affect your health and your future, your only hope is medical procedures and pharmaceutical drugs.

You are not powerless and you are not a victim. The health or disease you are experiencing today is largely the result of the diet and lifestyle decisions you've made in the past.

If you abuse your body, it is going to break down sooner, but if you take care of your body it will work better and you will increase your odds of health, healing, and long life. Today's choices affect tomorrow's health.

Your choices matter!

Be willing to do whatever it takes.

Once you have accepted responsibility for your health, the next step is being willing to do whatever it takes to get well, which means being willing to turn your life upside down, to change everything. If restoring my health meant getting as close to nature as possible by sleeping in the woods in a tent, I was willing to do it.

If it meant trekking out into the wilderness for a 40-day water fast like Jesus, I was willing to do it.

Fortunately, I didn't have to resort to either of those two things, but they were on my radar. I became a detective, determined to identify and eliminate anything in my life that may have contributed to my disease. I stopped eating to satisfy my appetite and sensual cravings and began eating to feed my cells, restore my health, and save my life. I wasn't living to eat anymore; I was eating to live.

Most cancer patients have a strong will to live in the beginning, but unfortunately, most of them have also been convinced that "doing whatever it takes," "living strong," and "fighting cancer" just means suffering through brutal and destructive cancer treatments. Whether you do conventional treatments or not, the Beat Cancer Mindset means taking an active role in your health and healing, not solely relying on someone else to cure you. I radically changed my diet and lifestyle. I gave up all the unhealthy food I loved to eat. I did every natural, nontoxic therapy I could find and afford. I faced my fears, admitted my faults, changed the way I thought, reached out to God and asked for help, and forgave everyone who had hurt me.

This was a lot more work than showing up for chemo and having my doctor's permission to eat burgers, ice cream, and pizza, and not changing my life, but I knew I had to do it.

The difference between successful people and unsuccessful people is not motivation. Motivation is unpredictable and unreliable.

It is easy to be motivated when you've started something new and exciting, but when the excitement wears off so does the motivation, and lack of motivation becomes an excuse for inaction.

What keeps people going when their motivation is low is determination.

Determination is the force inside you that cannot be stopped, even when the storms of life come against you.

Determination is doing what you know needs to be done, whether or not you feel like it at the time.

During this process, I became acutely aware of the spirit-mind-body connection as it relates to health and realized that not only did, I need to change my diet and lifestyle, but I also needed to change the way I was thinking.

My perspective on cancer is different from most. I don't see cancer as something to be fought or killed; I see it as something to be healed. There is a battle involved in healing cancer, but it's not so much a battle in the body as it is a battle in the mind. To heal your body, you must first win the battle in your mind.

Changing your thoughts will change your life.

When I caught myself thinking negatively, I chose to think positively. I chose to speak life out of my mouth and not allow outside influences, fear, and doubt to sway me.

When you think and speak this way, you empower your creative subconscious mind to assist you in the process, and you find supernatural strength to do things you never thought you could.

Your conscious mind and subconscious mind are powerful. Your beliefs are powerful. Patients who believe the treatment will help them often respond better than those who don't.

The placebo effect is real.

In my experience patients who go through the motions of treatment and therapies to appease those around them but don't believe they can get well rarely do. They subliminally sabotage the process and often make impulsive, irrational, emotion-based decisions that are not conducive to healing. When a doctor tells a patient, they are going to die in a matter of months, it can become a self-fulfilling prophecy.

They often lose all hope and stop trying to live. They believe they are going to die and they usually do, as predicted.

This is eerily not unlike a hex or a curse. No doctor has the authority to dictate the end of your life unless you give it to them.

They do not know when you will die. They are just lumping you into a statistical group based on your age, cancer type, stage, and other factors.

Your thoughts and beliefs create your life, your health, and your future. And when faced with a terminal prognosis, you have a choice of how to process that information. You can choose to believe it, or you can choose to reject it and become determined to prove your doctor wrong.

It's okay to accept a diagnosis, assuming it has been validated by several sources, but you don't have to accept a prognosis that you're going to die in a certain amount of time because a doctor or a statistic said so. Defy the odds and be the exception.

Take massive action.

The third characteristic of successful survivors is massive action.

Minimal action typically produces minimal results, but massive action produces massive results. Massive Action is radical action.

It's going against the grain. It's swimming upstream when everyone else is floating downstream. It's the action that draws jealousy and criticism from others. Humans by nature are resistant to change and tend to have a "crab mentality."

If you put crabs in a bucket and one tries to escape, the other crabs will pull it back down. In the same way, people often pull each other down out of envy, spite, or competitiveness.

Massive Action may appear crazy to people around you and they may try to talk you out of it like they did me, but don't let them. Massive Action is facing your flaws, faults, and fears, changing your whole life, getting rid of everything that might be keeping you sick, and replacing disease promoters with health promoters.

Sometimes small changes can produce big results. I love when that happens. But if that's what you're hoping for, your hope is in the wrong place because your hope is for a quick fix.

That's not the Beat Cancer Mindset. That's the Magic Bullet Mindset. And the conventional and alternative cancer industries are both full of people ready to take advantage of anyone looking for a shortcut.

You didn't get cancer overnight and you aren't going to get rid of it overnight. There is no miracle cure or magic bullet. Long-term healing requires massive action and a total life change. Point your ship toward Healthy Island and stay the course.

I've seen many cancer patients experience dramatic turnarounds in their health and have tumors shrink and even disappear in as little as 30 to 90 days using nutrition and nontoxic therapies, but I've also seen some of them become lazy and complacent and slide back into their old unhealthy habits.

Then cancer comes back. The first two years after a cancer diagnosis are the most critical. This is when cancer is most likely to return or spread. Two years of hard-core healthy living is an ideal short-term target, and beyond that, to stay healthy long-term, you have to make your health a priority for life.

Every day of your life is a page in your story. Your thoughts, decisions, and actions each day write your story. Take massive action to change your life and be 100 percent committed to the process. 100 percent is easy. 99 percent is hard.

Make plans for the future.

Document every detail of your cancer journey. Journal. Do a video diary. Plan on being well and document what you're doing so you can use what you've learned to help other people once you are well.

You need a future goal to work toward, and making plans for the future is very important. The spirit-mind-body connection is a mystery, but something powerful happens when you plan for the future.

You're planning to live. You're sending signals of life to your body. Don't be afraid to make plans for the future. I know the default response is, "Well, I don't know if I'll be here in a year or two years . . ." Instead of thinking that way, plan on living a long life. Sketch out your life goals, write down the things you want to accomplish, and keep those goals in front of you and start working toward them. Making plans for the future is so important. When I was diagnosed, I didn't have children and I wanted to have a family.

I wanted to be a dad. The decision to start a family three months after being diagnosed was a huge risk, but it took my focus off cancer, strengthened my will to live, and brought a new dimension of purpose into my life. If Micah and I had agreed not to have children for fear of an unknown future, we would not have our two beautiful daughters, the greatest joys in our life.

Enjoy your life and the process.

Don't let fear and worry steal your joy. Decide to live in the present and enjoy your life right now. Depression suppresses your immune system. If you're depressed, fearful, anxious, or worried, it makes you more vulnerable to cancer. Instead focus on things that bring you to hope, optimism, encouragement, and joy. Start living your life, really living. There's an organization for young adult cancer patients called Stupid Cancer and I love their slogan, which is "Get Busy Living."

Now is the time to live. There are a thousand different ways you could die besides cancer. You could die in a car wreck. You could trip and hit your head on the pavement. You could choke on a peppermint. There's no point in letting cancer paralyze you into depression and inaction. Start doing things you've always wanted to do. Get out there. Live your life. Do fun stuff. Do some skydiving, mountain climbing, and bull riding like it says in the Tim McGraw song "Live Like You Were Dying." Commit to enjoying your life and enjoying the process. And Get Busy Living!

Even if some of these changes are difficult for you, like quitting smoking, giving up your favourite unhealthy foods, or eating vegetables you've never liked, you've got to keep your perspective because there are way worse things than vegetables. And when you get well, you can look back and know it was all worth it.

This is a new chapter, a new season in life, a new adventure that should be dominated by gratitude.

Gratitude is the secret to happiness.

Count your blessings every day.

Don't focus on what you don't have. Focus on what you do have. Don't focus on what you can't do. Focus on what you can do. Cancer cut a dividing line in your life.

If you're focused on the past, longing for the days before cancer and wishing things were the way they used to be, you will only make yourself more miserable. What you focus on expands.

Focus on joy, happiness, love, and gratitude and they will increase in your life.

Focus on the present and on the things, you can do today to improve your health and make your life better.

In 2004 I was struggling to build a real estate business, barely making ends meet, and living in a tiny house, and I had cancer.

I had every reason to be negative, bitter, and angry. But I learned how to exercise gratitude, how to be thankful, how to focus on all the good things in my life instead of the bad, and how to be happy in my most difficult season of life. And although I would rather not go through cancer again, I know with absolute certainty that what it taught me changed me for the better. The worst thing that ever happened to me has made my life more fulfilling than I could ever have imagined.

That's the Cancer Mindset.

Volume 4: How to Starve Cancer

No meal offers 100% immunity against cancer. When a person includes cancer-fighting foods in their diet, their chance of getting the disease may be reduced. The greatest meals for preventing cancer are examined in this volume along with the research that backs up these assertions.

Apple

Apples are among the foods that naturally contain substances with powerful anticancer effects. Apples have anticancer qualities that might help prevent infections, heart disease, and inflammation.

The adage "one apple a day keeps the doctor away" is accurate. Polyphenols found in apples have intriguing anticancer effects.

Plant-based substances called polyphenols may guard against infections, cardiovascular disease, and inflammation. According to certain studies, polyphenols can combat tumours and prevent cancer.

For instance, the polyphenol phloretin inhibits the glucose transporter 2 (GLUT2) protein, which is involved in the progression of cancer cells.

Berries

Berries are a good source of dietary fibre, vitamins, and minerals. Berries' antioxidant qualities and possible health advantages have piqued scientists' curiosity.

According to one research, the molecule found in blackberries called anthocyanin decreases biomarkers for colon cancer.

Another research shows that blueberries' anti-inflammatory properties may stop the development of breast cancer tumors in mice.

Cruciferous plants

Cruciferous vegetables like broccoli, cauliflower, and kale are rich in healthy minerals including manganese, and vitamins K, and C.

Additionally, sulforaphane, a plant chemical having anticancer characteristics, is found in cruciferous vegetables.

According to one research, sulforaphane greatly slows the development of colon cancer cells and promotes cell death.

Sulforaphane and genistein, a substance found in soybeans, have been shown in another research to greatly reduce the growth and size of breast cancer tumours. Additionally, histone deacetylase, an enzyme linked to the emergence of cancer, is inhibited by sulforaphane.

According to one study, cruciferous veggies should be consumed three to five times a week for the highest cancer-prevention benefits.

Carrots

High levels of beta-carotene found in carrots may help to avoid certain cancers. Vitamin K, vitamin A, and antioxidants are among the many vital elements found in carrots.

Additionally, carrots have a lot of beta-carotene, which gives them their distinctive orange hue.

According to recent research, beta-carotene is essential for immune system support and may shield against several cancers.

According to an analysis of eight research, beta-carotene may lower the incidence of breast and prostate cancer.

Large fish

Salmon, mackerel, and anchovies are examples of fatty fish that are full of critical nutrients including vitamin B, potassium, and omega-3 fatty acids.

According to one research, those who consume more freshwater fish in their diets had a 53% reduced chance of developing colon cancer than those who consume less of it.

Another research discovered a relationship between fish oil intake in later life and a noticeably decreased risk for prostate cancer.

Last but not least, research including 68,109 individuals discovered that those who took fish oil supplements at least four times per week had a 63 percent lower risk of colon cancer than those who did not.

Medicines and Dietary Supplements

Even if the items on the above list are commonplace and easily accessible, some individuals may not want to significantly alter their diet or way of life. In this instance, a wide variety of vitamins and drugs with anticancer ingredients are readily accessible.

The anti-cancer qualities of vitamins A, C, and E are well known, and they may be found as supplements in most large food shops. The majority of the plant-based substances mentioned in this volume, including phloretin, anthocyanin, and sulforaphane, are pills.

Some individuals may see a reduction in their risk of developing cancer after using over-the-counter drugs like aspirin and ibuprofen.

Before beginning a new medicine or supplement regimen, always see a doctor.

Volume 5: Restoring Your Immune System

Our bodies don't have a single immune system, despite common perceptions. According to Cara Anselmo, a clinical dietitian nutritionist at Memorial Sloan Kettering Cancer Center, the immune system is made up of several organs, cells, and proteins that cooperate to ward against illnesses. Some cancer therapies might decrease an individual's immune system, making it difficult for their body to effectively fight against infection.

But even for them, according to Ms. Anselmo, the objective is not to accelerate quickly. Whether you have cancer or not, it's important to maintain a healthy balance in your immune system. Maintaining healthy behaviors will keep your body's systems running smoothly. Wintertime is a crucial time because viruses are more likely to spread indoors.

Think of the word "immune system" as being replaced with "a healthy body," advises Ms. Anselmo. Here are some of her tips for boosting your resistance.

Organize your plate.

There is no one magic meal that will keep your immunity in check, just as there is no one element to the immune system (sorry!). However, a lot of meals may be beneficial. Everyone has heard how vitamin C works to fight off diseases like colds. There are many reasons why this vitamin deserves particular mention: Since vitamin C is an antioxidant, it counteracts the destructive, cell-destroying chemicals known as free radicals. Additionally, it promotes the development of antibodies and white blood cells, both of which work to fight infection. Vitamin C cannot be produced by the body; it is only found in foods.

However, it does not obligate you to consume one orange each day. In addition, foods like tomatoes, bell peppers, and strawberries, to mention a few, contain vitamin C. Although consuming foods high in vitamin C is necessary, most individuals don't need to take vitamin C supplements.

Numerous additional nutrients help maintain a strong immune system. Systemic inflammation may be decreased by eating a diet high in cruciferous vegetables, such as broccoli, cauliflower, kale, and Brussels sprouts. The anti-inflammatory properties of allium vegetables including garlic, scallions, and onion are similar. The nutritional content of these items is the same whether you eat them cooked or raw. Protein is also crucial. Proteins from both animals and plants are used to create new cells and repair damaged tissue, acting as an offensive and defensive weapon against invading organisms.

2. Drink plenty of water.

Our mucous membranes are one line of protection against illness, according to Ms. Anselmo. "People concentrate so much on food, and certainly, diet is essential," she adds. To operate at their optimum, water keeps them wet. These shielding liners may be found in your nose, mouth, and eyes, and they function like bouncers at a club to keep away intruders. However, did you know that several bodily parts, like the stomach and the female and male reproductive systems, have mucous membranes covering them as well? The advice to consume eight glasses of water each day may not be required. You may get specialized advice from your professional dietitian or nutritionist.

3. Avoid depending on supplements.

They are not intended to substitute a balanced diet. However, consult your medical team before taking any supplements since some of them, like vitamin D (more on that later), may prevent or remedy certain nutritional deficits. Just remember to not conflate "natural" with "safe." As with any oral vitamin, mineral, herbal, or another supplement, those touted for "raising immunity" may have more negative effects than positive ones, according to Ms. Anselmo.

4. Verify your vitamin D intake.

Without a doubt: It helps create strength, as we are aware. But vitamin D also maintains the health of T cells and macrophages, two kinds of cells that fight illness. Humans get this mineral by exposure to sunlight rather than through eating. Even if you follow the cleanest diet known to man, Ms. Anselmo warns, you could not receive enough vitamin D. Even milk, which we have all been told is a wonderful source, is insufficient.

You could require a supplement since many people are unfortunately vitamin D deficient due to the long, chilly winters. Your levels may be examined by your doctor via a blood test.

what is in your refrigerator

5. Continue going.

Your lungs and airways may become free of microorganisms if you exercise. Additionally, it reduces the production of stress hormones, which is important as too much stress might impair immunity. You don't have to put forth a lot of effort to get the rewards. Walking is a self-paced activity that doesn't need any special equipment, according to Ms. Anselmo. She also suggests doing exercises that increase your strength, like yoga or lifting weights. Ms. Anselmo gives the following guidance after your doctor has given the all-clear for you to begin a new workout routine: Start slowly, gradually increase the intensity and frequency, and pay attention to your body.

6. Make sleep a priority.

We often believe that we can go without sleep if we follow a healthy diet and exercise regimen, Ms. Anselmo explains. But sleep is quite important. The immune system is actively producing proteins that bolster the body's viral defenses while we sleep. She advises that taking daytime naps to catch up is OK, but try to limit them to no more than 30 minutes to avoid changing your circadian cycle.

This page was left blank intentionally

Volume 6: Spiritual Healing

A cancer diagnosis is a life-changing event that causes worry, anxiety, and bewilderment. And the long, arduous fight that comes after hearing the dreadful words, "You have cancer," requires all of the strength and bravery you possess. Your daily routine is consumed by many hours of chemotherapy, radiation, and surgery, and the tranquillity you once knew vanishes.

Perhaps it seems like everyone else's life is going along just fine while yours seems to be stagnant. Or you may come to feel completely alone in this titanic conflict. You may be reminded that God is the One who cares about what you're going through and who will always be there for you by reading or performing prayers for cancer.

For those who practice a religion, faith is essential to every facet of life. But amid a severe sickness, it takes on much more significance. When all you want to do is fall apart, it keeps you together. And because of your faith, you can wield the potent instrument of prayer. You may reach the universe's creator directly, day or night, by offering a prayer for the ill.

No matter what stage of your cancer journey you're in, let these cancer prayers renew your spirit and heal your soul in a way that only God's presence can. And while you continue to struggle, let your source of hope be healing prayers.

A BLESSING PRAYER

Please, Lord, I pray for grace so that I may overcome the difficulties I face. You are aware that I want to live. I don't want my body to alter, you know. I don't want to become ill; you know. You also understand why I must take on this endeavour and go down this terrifying road. I wish to keep it away. I want medical professionals to correct the diagnosis for me. My life should go back to how it was. I do not comprehend. But I am certain that You will lead me if I place my hand in Yours. You'll inspire me with bravery. You'll give me solace. I beg Your forgiveness right now and always. Amen.

- In the Notre Dame Book of Prayer, Anne Thompson

A BLESSING FOR COURAGE

But if it should be God's Holy Will that I endure this illness, give me the courage and fortitude to accept these hardships from God's loving hand with patience and resignation, because he knows what is best for the salvation of my soul. God knows what is best for me.

A BLESSING FOR RECOVERY

We are grateful to you, Heavenly Father, for the way you accompany us through our darkest valleys. We are grateful that you shared our suffering by sending your Son to experience life, death, and all in between for us. Your Word declares that you are close to the grieving and that you deliver the downcast. Bring us nearer to you, O Prince of Peace, as we seek the meaning of life. We appreciate your kindness and beg for your recovery so that you may restore the bodies of those who endure the physical anguish and psychological stress caused by cancer. Lord, we confidently beg for discoveries that will result in improved therapies and the ultimate elimination of the havoc brought on by cancer. As you carry out your will, may you be given all the praise? Amen, in the powerful name of Jesus.

- from The Notre Dame Book of Prayer, Ian Lightcap

BLESSING FOR PEACE

Don't worry or fret. Pray instead of worrying. Let God know your concerns by forming them into praises and pleas in your prayers. Before you realize it, a feeling of God's completeness, of everything working out for the best, will settle over you. What occurs when Christ takes worry's place at the heart of your life is amazing.

— Philippians letter of Paul, verse seven The Translation

A BLESSING FOR SUCCESS

Lord, I'm exhausted and unsure of when my life's "marathon" will come to a finish. To escape this ordeal, I feel as if I have been running for ages. Help me to stop attempting to flee my agony and instead run the race you have put before me with endurance. I am aware that I will finally triumph over my struggles in life because of you. I am aware that nothing in this world can sever my connection to your unwavering love. Please shower me with your love today and give me the stamina to go through this ordeal. I appreciate your unending devotion to me. And thank you for my everlasting crown of delight in your Kingdom!

- Adrien Rogers (Gwen Smith)